Keto OMAD Diet

A Beginner's Step-by-Step Guide to Getting Started, with Sample Recipes and a Meal Plan

copyright © 2023 Larry Jamesonn

All rights reserved No part of this book may be reproduced, or stored in a retrieval system, or transmitted in any form or by any means, electronic, mechanical, photocopying, recording, or otherwise, without express written permission of the publisher.

Disclaimer

By reading this disclaimer, you are accepting the terms of the disclaimer in full. If you disagree with this disclaimer, please do not read the guide.

All of the content within this guide is provided for informational and educational purposes only, and should not be accepted as independent medical or other professional advice. The author is not a doctor, physician, nurse, mental health provider, or registered nutritionist/dietician. Therefore, using and reading this guide does not establish any form of a physician-patient relationship.

Always consult with a physician or another qualified health provider with any issues or questions you might have regarding any sort of medical condition. Do not ever disregard any qualified professional medical advice or delay seeking that advice because of anything you have read in this guide. The information in this guide is not intended to be any sort of medical advice and should not be used in lieu of any medical advice by a licensed and qualified medical professional.

The information in this guide has been compiled from a variety of known sources. However, the author cannot attest to or guarantee the accuracy of each source and thus should not be held liable for any errors or omissions.

You acknowledge that the publisher of this guide will not be held liable for any loss or damage of any kind incurred as a result of this guide or the reliance on any information provided within this guide. You acknowledge and agree that you assume all risk and responsibility for any action you undertake in response to the information in this guide.

Using this guide does not guarantee any particular result (e.g., weight loss or a cure). By reading this guide, you acknowledge that there are no guarantees to any specific outcome or results you can expect.

All product names, diet plans, or names used in this guide are for identification purposes only and are the property of their respective owners. The use of these names does not imply endorsement. All other trademarks cited herein are the property of their respective owners.

Where applicable, this guide is not intended to be a substitute for the original work of this diet plan and is, at most, a supplement to the original work for this diet plan and never a direct substitute. This guide is a personal expression of the facts of that diet plan.

Where applicable, persons shown in the cover images are stock photography models and the publisher has obtained the rights to use the images through license agreements with third-party stock image companies.

Table of Contents

Introduction	**8**
Everything About Keto OMAD Diet	**10**
The Ketogenic Diet	10
What Is OMAD?	13
The Keto OMAD Diet	15
Principles of Keto OMAD Diet	16
Health Benefits of the Keto OMAD Diet	19
Pros and Cons	**22**
Pros of the Keto OMAD Diet	22
Cons of the Keto OMAD Diet	23
5 Step-Guide to Get Started with the Keto OMAD Diet	**26**
Step 1: Educate Yourself about the Keto OMAD Diet	26
Step 2: Determine Your Macronutrient Ratios	27
Step 3: Plan Your Meals Strategically	27
Step 4: Ease into Intermittent Fasting	28
Step 5: Monitor Your Progress and Make Adjustments	28
Foods to Eat	29
Foods to Avoid	33
Sample Recipes	**38**
Bacon-Wrapped Chicken Thighs	39
Salmon with Asparagus	40
Cauliflower Fried Rice	41
Egg and Avocado Salad Lettuce Wraps	43
Zucchini Noodles with Pesto and Grilled Chicken	44
Steak with Creamy Garlic Mushrooms	45
Taco Stuffed Bell Peppers	46
Creamy Spinach and Feta Stuffed Chicken	48
Cauliflower Crust Pizza	49
Shrimp Stir-Fry	51

Mediterranean Salad Paired with Charbroiled Chicken	53
Zucchini and Bacon Egg Muffins	55
Lemon Garlic Shrimp Skewers	56
Caprese Stuffed Portobello Mushrooms	57
Chocolate Avocado Mousse	59
7-Day Meal Plan	**60**
Conclusion	**62**
FAQs	**66**
Resources and Helpful Links	**68**

Introduction

According to research, people in the past ate only once or twice, at the most, a day, and this was enough to sustain them throughout the day. They didn't necessarily had a feast, but they ate what their body needed to survive and accomplished what needed to be done for the day.

This practice of one meal a day is believed to be a good way for people to maintain good weight and avoid unnecessary eating, which usually lead to several diseases like diabetes and excessive weight gain. This is why Keto OMAD Diet has gotten popular nowadays, as it provides an alternative yet effective dietary practice for those who need it.

The Keto OMAD Diet combines two proven methods - the ketogenic diet and intermittent fasting. Keto is a low-carb, high-fat diet that promotes ketosis, where the body burns fat for fuel. Intermittent fasting involves restricting the eating window to a few hours a day, followed by a fasting period. This approach accelerates fat-burning and weight loss.

By adopting the Keto OMAD Diet, individuals can leverage the synergistic effects of these two powerful strategies. Not only does it facilitate rapid weight loss, but it also provides a myriad of additional benefits. From increased mental clarity and improved energy levels to better blood sugar control and enhanced metabolic health, the Keto OMAD Diet offers a comprehensive approach to transforming both your body and mind.

Imagine waking up each day with endless energy, feeling confident and in control of your body. The Keto OMAD Diet turns these dreams into reality. This guide provides a deep understanding of the principles behind the diet and how to incorporate it into your routine. You'll learn about optimal macronutrient ratios, tasty meal ideas, and practical strategies for sustainable success.

In this Guide, we will talk about the following:

- What is the Keto OMAD Diet?
- The Ketogenic Diet and What is OMAD?
- Principles and Health Benefits of the Keto OMAD Diet
- 5-Step Guide to Get Started with The Keto OMAD Diet
- Foods to Eat and To Avoid with the Keto OMAD Diet
- Sample Recipes and Meal Plan

Are you tired of trying different diets that promise remarkable results but fail to deliver? Are you ready to take control of your health and achieve your weight loss goals efficiently? If so, then the Keto OMAD Diet is here to revolutionize the way you approach your nutrition and lifestyle. By understanding how this powerful combination of ketogenic eating and intermittent fasting can work wonders for your body, you'll be equipped with the tools needed to unlock your true potential.

Keep reading as we delve into the fundamentals of the Keto OMAD Diet, exploring its history, scientific basis, and the principles that make it a powerful tool for weight loss and overall well-being. Get ready to unlock the secrets to a healthier, fitter you!

Keto OMAD Diet 101: What Is It?

The Ketogenic Diet

The ketogenic diet is a low-carbohydrate, high-fat eating plan that has gained popularity for its potential health benefits. It entails lowering carbohydrate intake and substituting healthy fats for them in order to put the body into a metabolic condition known as ketosis.

In a typical Western diet, the primary source of energy comes from carbohydrates. However, in the ketogenic diet, carb intake is significantly limited, usually to less than 50 grams per day or about 5-10% of total calories. This restriction forces the body to seek an alternative fuel source.

When carbohydrate intake is restricted, the body starts breaking down stored fat into molecules called ketones. Ketones are then used as a fuel source by the body's cells, including the brain. This process of relying on fat for energy instead of glucose is known as ketosis.

The macronutrient ratios of the ketogenic diet typically involve:

- High Fat: About 70-75% of daily calorie intake comes from healthy fats such as avocados, nuts, seeds, olive oil, coconut oil, and fatty fish.
- Moderate Protein: Approximately 20-25% of daily calories are derived from sources like poultry, lean meats, eggs, and dairy products.
- Low Carbohydrate: Carbohydrate intake is limited to around 5-10% of total calorie intake and mostly comes from non-starchy vegetables and small amounts of berries.

By following this eating pattern, individuals on the ketogenic diet aim to achieve several potential benefits, including:

- Weight Loss: The ketogenic diet aids in weight loss by reducing carbohydrate intake, resulting in increased fat burning and decreased appetite. When following the diet, the body enters a state of ketosis, where it uses stored fat as its primary fuel source. This promotes weight loss and can be an effective strategy for those looking to shed pounds.
- Improved Blood Sugar Control: Restricting carbohydrates on the ketogenic diet improves blood sugar control, benefiting individuals with diabetes or insulin resistance. By minimizing carbohydrate intake, the body experiences fewer spikes in blood sugar levels, reducing the need for excess insulin production.

This can lead to better glycemic control and improved overall health.

- Enhanced Mental Clarity: When in ketosis, individuals may experience enhanced mental clarity and focus. This is attributed to the brain's utilization of ketones as a fuel source, which provides a stable energy supply without the fluctuations associated with glucose metabolism. Many people find this aspect of the ketogenic diet beneficial for cognitive function and productivity.
- Increased Energy Levels: Individuals on the ketogenic diet may experience increased energy levels and sustained endurance throughout the day. As the body becomes efficient at utilizing fat for energy, it can provide a steady and reliable source of fuel, resulting in improved vitality and reduced fatigue. This can be particularly beneficial for athletes or those with demanding daily routines.

Please consult a healthcare professional or registered dietitian before starting the ketogenic diet, as it may not be suitable for everyone. It's important to stay hydrated and incorporate nutrient-dense foods for a safe and effective ketogenic diet.

Remember, individual results and experiences may vary, so it's important to listen to your body and make adjustments as needed while on the ketogenic diet.

What Is OMAD?

OMAD, which stands for "One Meal a Day," is a form of intermittent fasting where an individual consumes all of their daily caloric intake within a single meal, typically lasting for about an hour. The rest of the day is spent in a fasting state, consuming no additional calories.

With OMAD, individuals choose a specific time window, usually in the evening, to have their one meal. During this meal, they aim to meet their nutritional needs by including a balanced combination of proteins, carbohydrates, and healthy fats. However, it is essential to prioritize nutrient-dense foods to ensure adequate nourishment.

OMAD has gained popularity due to its simplicity and potential benefits. Here are some key aspects of OMAD:

1. Simplicity: OMAD simplifies meal planning and eliminates the need for frequent food preparation throughout the day. It allows individuals to focus on a single, satisfying meal, reducing the time spent on eating-related activities.

2. Caloric Restriction: By consuming only one meal a day, OMAD naturally restricts caloric intake. This can create a calorie deficit, potentially leading to weight loss over time. However, it is crucial to ensure that a single meal provides enough nutrients to support overall health.

3. Autophagy and Metabolic Adaptation: Extended periods of fasting, such as those experienced with OMAD, can stimulate autophagy—a cellular process that helps remove damaged cells and promote cellular repair. Additionally, OMAD can lead to metabolic adaptations, such as improved insulin sensitivity and fat-burning capacity.

4. Potential Challenges: OMAD may not be suitable for everyone, as it can be challenging to consume all the necessary nutrients within a single meal. It may also require adjustment to fit individual lifestyles and social situations. Additionally, individuals with certain health conditions or dietary restrictions should consult with a healthcare professional before adopting OMAD.

5. Personalization: OMAD can be customized to fit individual preferences. Some individuals choose to follow OMAD daily, while others adopt it a few times per week. It's important to find a schedule that works best for your lifestyle and supports your health goals.

As with any significant dietary change, it's recommended to consult with a healthcare professional or registered dietitian before starting OMAD, especially if you have underlying health conditions or nutritional needs.

In summary, OMAD is a form of intermittent fasting where individuals consume all their daily caloric intake within a single meal. It simplifies meal planning, and promotes potential benefits like caloric restriction and metabolic adaptations, but may pose challenges in meeting nutritional needs. Personalization and professional guidance are essential when considering OMAD as a dietary approach.

The Keto OMAD Diet

The Keto OMAD Diet is a combination of two popular dietary approaches: the ketogenic diet and intermittent fasting, particularly the one-meal-a-day diet. The ketogenic diet involves consuming a high-fat, moderate-protein, and low-carbohydrate diet to induce a metabolic state called ketosis, where the body burns fat for fuel instead of carbohydrates. Intermittent fasting, on the other hand, involves cycling between periods of eating and fasting.

The Keto OMAD Diet has gained significant popularity due to its effectiveness in achieving weight loss goals. Combining the principles of the ketogenic diet and intermittent fasting, it provides a powerful tool for those looking to shed excess pounds. The low-carb, high-fat nature of the diet helps suppress appetite and optimize fat burning, while intermittent fasting further enhances weight loss by promoting a longer fasting period and improving insulin sensitivity.

Many individuals who have followed the Keto OMAD Diet have reported significant weight loss results. By restricting carbohydrate intake and incorporating periods of fasting, the body is encouraged to tap into its fat stores for energy, leading to accelerated fat loss. Additionally, the diet's focus on nutrient-dense, whole foods promotes overall health and can contribute to sustained weight management.

Principles of Keto OMAD Diet

The Keto OMAD (One Meal A Day) diet combines the principles of the ketogenic diet with intermittent fasting to promote weight loss, fat burning, and other health benefits. Here are the key principles of the Keto OMAD diet:

1. Ketogenic Diet: The foundation of the Keto OMAD diet is the ketogenic eating plan. It involves consuming a high-fat, moderate-protein, and low-carbohydrate diet. The goal is to induce a state of ketosis, where the body primarily uses fat for fuel instead of carbohydrates.

2. One Meal A Day: The Keto OMAD diet incorporates intermittent fasting by restricting the eating window to one meal per day. This involves fasting for approximately 23 hours and consuming all daily calories within a limited time frame, typically around 1 hour.

3. Macronutrient Ratios: Following the ketogenic principles, the Keto OMAD diet emphasizes specific macronutrient ratios. The typical breakdown is around

70-75% of calories from fat, 20-25% from protein, and 5-10% from carbohydrates. This ratio helps the body enter and maintain ketosis.

4. Limit Carbohydrate Intake: To achieve and sustain ketosis, carbohydrate intake should be restricted. The Keto OMAD diet recommends consuming no more than 20-50 grams of net carbs per day. This restriction forces the body to rely on fat as its primary energy source.

5. Focus on Healthy Fats: Healthy fats play a crucial role in the Keto OMAD diet. Foods rich in monounsaturated fats (like avocados, olive oil, and nuts), saturated fats (from sources like coconut oil and grass-fed butter), and omega-3 fatty acids (found in fatty fish and flaxseeds) are encouraged.

6. Adequate Protein Intake: While the Keto OMAD diet is high in fat, it also requires a moderate intake of protein. Protein helps with muscle maintenance and satiety. Consuming lean sources of protein, such as poultry, fish, and tofu, is recommended.

7. Hydration: Staying properly hydrated is essential for the Keto OMAD diet. It's crucial to drink sufficient water throughout the day to prevent dehydration and support bodily functions. Adding electrolytes can also

help maintain electrolyte balance, especially in the early stages of ketosis.

8. Nutrient-Dense Foods: To ensure adequate nutrient intake, it's important to focus on nutrient-dense foods within one meal. Incorporate a variety of non-starchy vegetables, leafy greens, and low-sugar fruits to provide essential vitamins and minerals.

9. Monitoring Ketone Levels: Regularly monitoring ketone levels using urine strips or blood tests can help ensure that the body is in a state of ketosis. This provides insight into dietary adjustments and helps track progress.

10. Individualization and Consultation: It's important to remember that the Keto OMAD diet may not be suitable for everyone. Consulting with a healthcare professional or registered dietitian is recommended, especially for those with underlying health conditions or specific dietary needs.

By combining the principles of the ketogenic diet with intermittent fasting, the Keto OMAD diet can be an effective way to support weight loss and overall health. It's essential to consider individual needs and consult with a healthcare professional when considering making dietary changes. Additionally, following the key principles of this approach is recommended for optimal results.

Health Benefits of the Keto OMAD Diet

The Keto OMAD (One Meal a Day) diet is known for its potential health benefits. While further research is needed to fully understand the effects, some of the reported health benefits include:

- Weight loss: The combination of the ketogenic and OMAD (One Meal a Day) approaches can lead to enhanced weight loss for individuals. This is achieved by promoting fat burning through ketosis and reducing overall calorie intake due to the limited eating window. The synergistic effect of these strategies can expedite the weight loss process.
- Improved body composition: The Keto OMAD diet has the potential to improve body composition by reducing body fat while preserving lean muscle mass. Through the combination of the ketogenic state and the disciplined eating pattern, individuals can optimize fat loss while minimizing muscle breakdown, resulting in a more desirable body composition.
- Better insulin sensitivity and blood sugar regulation: The Keto OMAD diet has the potential to improve insulin sensitivity and regulate blood sugar levels by limiting carbohydrate intake. This dietary approach encourages the body to rely on fat for fuel, reducing the need for insulin secretion and promoting stable

blood sugar levels, which can be beneficial for individuals with insulin resistance or diabetes.
- Enhanced heart health: Preliminary studies indicate that the Keto OMAD diet may have favorable impacts on cardiovascular health markers, including blood pressure, cholesterol levels, and triglycerides. These findings suggest that this dietary approach could potentially contribute to enhanced heart health and reduce the risk of cardiovascular diseases when followed under proper guidance and supervision.
- Increased metabolic flexibility: The Keto OMAD diet has shown potential in increasing metabolic flexibility, enabling the body to efficiently switch between utilizing carbohydrates and fats as fuel sources. By restricting carbohydrate intake and promoting fat adaptation, this dietary approach encourages the body to become more adept at utilizing stored fat for energy. This enhanced metabolic flexibility may have numerous benefits, including improved endurance, stable energy levels, and enhanced weight management.
- Neuroprotective properties: The production of ketones during the Keto OMAD diet has been linked to potential neuroprotective properties, suggesting that it may have benefits in safeguarding and enhancing brain health. Ketones serve as an alternative energy source for the brain, potentially improving cognitive function

and offering protection against neurodegenerative conditions. Further research is needed to fully understand and validate these findings.

It's important to note that individual responses to the Keto OMAD diet may vary, and these health benefits are not guaranteed for everyone. It's always recommended to consult with a healthcare professional or registered dietitian before making any significant changes to your diet.

Pros and Cons

The Keto OMAD diet can be a great option for those looking to lose weight, regulate blood sugar levels, and optimize health. However, as with any dietary intervention, there are both pros and cons to consider before starting.

Pros of the Keto OMAD Diet

Incorporating the principles of the Keto OMAD diet can offer several advantages, which may include:

- Simplicity: Following the Keto OMAD diet involves eating only one meal a day, which can simplify meal planning and preparation.
- Time-saving: With only one meal to focus on, the Keto OMAD diet can save time in meal preparation, allowing individuals to have more time for other activities.
- Potential cost savings: Eating one meal a day may lead to decreased food expenses, as there are fewer meals to purchase and prepare.
- Increased discipline: The Keto OMAD diet requires discipline and self-control, which can help individuals

develop a stronger sense of willpower and determination.
- Potential health benefits: The Keto OMAD diet has been associated with various health benefits, including weight loss, improved blood sugar control, and reduced inflammation.
- Flexibility: While the Keto OMAD diet has specific guidelines, it allows for flexibility in choosing the types of foods and recipes that align with the principles of the diet.
- Portion control: Eating only one meal a day can help individuals practice portion control and become more mindful of their eating habits.
- Potential metabolic benefits: The Keto OMAD diet may promote fat burning and improve insulin sensitivity, potentially leading to metabolic improvements.

Please keep in mind that the advantages of the Keto OMAD diet may vary from person to person, and it's important to consult with a healthcare professional or registered dietitian before starting any new diet plan.

Cons of the Keto OMAD Diet

The Keto OMAD diet, despite its benefits, does have several disadvantages. However, it is important to note that the benefits of this diet often outweigh these drawbacks. Here are some disadvantages of the Keto OMAD diet:

- Restrictive Nature: The Keto OMAD diet can be highly restrictive, as it involves consuming only one meal a day and following a strict ketogenic eating plan. This level of restriction may make it challenging for some individuals to adhere to the diet in the long term.
- Limited Food Choices: Following the Keto OMAD diet can limit food choices, especially when eating out or at social gatherings. It may be difficult to find suitable keto-friendly meals, which can make it more challenging to stick to the diet consistently.
- Potential Nutrient Deficiencies: The limited food options on the Keto OMAD diet can lead to potential nutrient deficiencies, particularly if individuals are not careful about including a wide variety of nutrient-rich foods in their single meal. Adequate planning and supplementation may be necessary to ensure all essential nutrients are obtained.
- Adverse Effects: Some individuals may experience adverse effects while following the Keto OMAD diet, such as low blood pressure, kidney stones, constipation, and an increased risk of heart disease. These risks should be taken into consideration before starting the diet, especially for individuals with certain health conditions.

- Lack of Flexibility: The Keto OMAD diet may lack flexibility compared to other eating plans. It can be challenging to adapt the diet to different schedules or specific dietary preferences, which may pose difficulties for some individuals.

It's important to consult with a healthcare professional or registered dietitian before starting any new diet plan, including the Keto OMAD diet. They can provide personalized advice and guidance based on individual needs and health conditions.

5 Step-Guide to Get Started with the Keto OMAD Diet

The Keto OMAD diet is a combination of the ketogenic diet and intermittent fasting, focusing on eating one meal per day. Here are 5 steps to help get started with the Keto OMAD diet:

Step 1: Educate Yourself about the Keto OMAD Diet

To get started with the Keto OMAD diet, you should educate yourself on how it works and its benefits. The Keto OMAD diet combines the ketogenic diet and intermittent fasting to promote weight loss and overall health. By consuming a high-fat, moderate protein, and low-carbohydrate diet, your body enters a state of ketosis, which burns fat for fuel.

Intermittent fasting then restricts the period for when you eat, allowing your body to fully enter ketosis and increase fat burning. This diet has been shown to improve insulin sensitivity, reduce inflammation, and improve brain function. Consult a healthcare professional or reputable sources to gather accurate information and proceed with caution.

Step 2: Determine Your Macronutrient Ratios

After researching, the next step is to determine your macronutrient ratios - the proportions of healthy fats, proteins, and carbohydrates you need daily. For the Keto OMAD diet, aim for approximately 70-75% of daily calories from healthy fats, 20-25% from protein, and only 5-10% from carbohydrates. These ratios may vary based on your needs and goals, so use an online keto calculator to determine specific ratios based on age, weight, height, gender, and activity level. Plan your meals accordingly and start seeing results with this effective weight-loss method.

Step 3: Plan Your Meals Strategically

The third step is to plan your meals strategically. Focus on high-quality, healthy fats as the primary source of energy such as avocados, nuts, seeds, olive oil, and coconut oil. These fats help keep you feeling full and satisfied throughout the day, which is crucial when consuming only one meal a day. Incorporate moderate amounts of protein from sources like eggs, poultry, fish, or tofu to prevent muscle loss.

Keep your carbohydrate intake extremely low by choosing non-starchy vegetables like leafy greens, cauliflower, and zucchini. These vegetables contain fiber and important vitamins and minerals while being low in carbs. By carefully planning your meals with these guidelines in mind, you can successfully transition to the Keto OMAD diet and reap its many benefits.

Step 4: Ease into Intermittent Fasting

To successfully follow the Keto OMAD diet, it is essential to gradually ease into intermittent fasting. This is achieved by slowly extending the fasting period each day. For instance, if you usually have breakfast at 8am, consider delaying it to 10 a.m. for a few days, then gradually increase fasting hours until you attain your desired one-hour eating window.

Remember to remain hydrated during the fasting period, and consume water, black coffee, or herbal tea. Intermittent fasting is a crucial aspect of the Keto OMAD diet, and it helps in boosting metabolism and reducing insulin levels. By adhering to this step, you can achieve the full benefits of the Keto OMAD diet.

Step 5: Monitor Your Progress and Make Adjustments

It's crucial to monitor your progress regularly and make necessary adjustments. The first step is to be mindful of your macronutrient intake and meal timing. Maintaining a proper balance of carbs, fats, and protein is key to achieving ketosis, the state where your body burns fat for energy. It's recommended to consume no more than 20-30 grams of net carbs per day, as carbs can disrupt ketosis.

Next, focus on establishing a regular one-meal-a-day eating pattern. This will help regulate your appetite and aid in weight loss. Keep track of your progress by using smartphone apps or journals to record your food intake, weight, and body measurements. Remember, if you encounter any difficulties or setbacks, consult a healthcare professional or certified nutritionist who can provide you with guidance and necessary adjustments to help you achieve your goals.

Remember, it's essential to listen to your body and prioritize your overall health. The Keto OMAD diet may not be suitable for everyone, especially those with specific medical conditions or dietary restrictions. Consult with a healthcare professional before starting any new diet or making significant changes to your eating habits.

By following these steps, you'll be well on your way to embracing the Keto OMAD diet and reaping its potential benefits. Good luck on your journey toward a healthier lifestyle!

Foods to Eat

When following the Keto OMAD diet, it's important to focus on eating nutrient-dense whole foods. Here are some of the best foods to include in your single meal each day:

1. **Lean proteins**: For a successful Keto OMAD diet, focus on lean proteins like chicken, turkey, beef, pork,

fish, and eggs to ensure you're getting essential amino acids for muscle growth and repair. These foods are low in carbs and high in fat, making them perfect for this diet plan. Aim to include various protein sources in your daily meals for optimal nutrition and satiety.

2. **Non-starchy vegetables**: For a Keto OMAD diet, make sure to pick non-starchy vegetables like spinach, kale, lettuce, broccoli, cauliflower, zucchini, and asparagus. These are great sources of fiber, vitamins, minerals, and antioxidants.

Consuming a variety of vegetables ensures you get the necessary nutrients while staying within your carb limit. Remember, the key to a successful keto diet is achieving and maintaining ketosis, and non-starchy veggies are essential in doing so.

3. **Healthy fats**: Include avocados, nuts like almonds and walnuts, and seeds such as chia and flax seeds in your Keto OMAD diet. These foods offer essential fatty acids, promote satiety, and aid in ketosis.

Olives are also an excellent source of healthy fats, making them an ideal addition to your eating plan. Incorporating these foods into your daily routine can help you achieve your weight loss and health goals while maintaining an enjoyable and satisfying eating experience.

4. **Full-fat dairy products**: Incorporate full-fat cheese, butter, heavy cream, and Greek yogurt into your Keto OMAD diet. These foods are rich in healthy fats and protein while being low in carbs, making them perfect for maintaining ketosis.

   Additionally, full-fat dairy products provide your body with essential vitamins and minerals such as calcium, vitamin D, and vitamin K2. Enjoy a variety of full-fat dairy options to stay satiated and healthy on your Keto OMAD journey.

5. **Low-carb fruits**: When following a Keto OMAD diet, it's important to be mindful of the foods you consume. Berries such as strawberries, blueberries, and raspberries are excellent low-carb options that are rich in antioxidants and can help with weight loss. One cup of strawberries contains only 8 grams of net carbs, whereas one cup of blueberries contains 17 grams.

   Meanwhile, raspberries contain just 5 grams per cup. These small, sweet treats can be enjoyed as a snack or added to a salad for a burst of flavor. Remember, moderation is key when including any fruit in a Keto OMAD meal plan.

6. **High-fiber foods**: For your Keto OMAD diet, incorporate chia seeds, flaxseeds, psyllium husk, and fiber-rich vegetables such as Brussels sprouts and

broccoli. These foods are crucial for maintaining a healthy digestive system and preventing constipation.

Not only do they provide essential nutrients, but their high fiber content helps keep you feeling full longer throughout the day. So, make sure to stock up on these fiber-packed foods to ensure a successful Keto OMAD diet.

7. **Healthy oils**: Healthy oils are a must-have when following a Keto OMAD diet. Opt for coconut oil, olive oil, and avocado oil as they contain healthy fats and aid in weight loss.

These plant-based oils can be used to flavor foods or added to your salad for an extra boost of nutrition. Additionally, these oils provide essential vitamins and minerals and can help regulate hormone levels.

8. **Condiments and spices**: For an extra flavor kick, add condiments and spices to your Keto OMAD meals. Spices like ginger, turmeric, and cumin are excellent additions as they have multiple health benefits and can be used in a variety of dishes.

Healthy condiments such as apple cider vinegar, balsamic vinegar, Dijon mustard, coconut aminos, and hot sauce are great for adding a zesty twist to your meals.

Remember, it's important to consult with a healthcare professional or registered dietitian before starting any new diet to ensure it aligns with your specific health needs and goals.

Foods to Avoid

Incorporating nutrient-rich foods is important when following the Keto OMAD diet, but it's also necessary to be aware of which foods should be limited or avoided. Here are some of the top food items that should be avoided on this eating plan:

1. **Processed carbohydrates**: When it comes to processed carbohydrates, it's best to steer clear of refined grains such as white bread, pasta, and rice. Additionally, be mindful of sugary cereals, cookies, and pastries, as they are not only high in carbohydrates but also have the potential to cause a rapid spike in blood sugar levels. By avoiding these types of processed carbs, you can make healthier dietary choices and maintain more stable blood sugar levels throughout the day.

2. **Sugary foods and beverages**: To maintain a state of ketosis and prevent energy crashes, it is highly recommended to steer clear of sugary foods and beverages. This includes not only soda, fruit juices, sports drinks, candy, and desserts, but also any other products that are laden with added sugars. By avoiding

these foods, you can ensure that your body stays in a fat-burning mode and experiences sustained energy levels throughout the day.

3. **High-carb fruits**: When following a low-carb or ketogenic diet, it is recommended to limit the consumption of high-sugar fruits like bananas, grapes, and pineapple. These fruits, while delicious and nutritious, contain a significant amount of carbohydrates that can potentially hinder the state of ketosis, which is essential for achieving the desired metabolic effects. By being mindful of the carbohydrate content in these fruits, you can better manage your intake and stay on track with your dietary goals.

4. **Starchy vegetables**: When it comes to starchy vegetables, it's advisable to minimize your intake of potatoes, corn, peas, and carrots. These particular veggies tend to be higher in carbohydrates compared to non-starchy alternatives, which may impact your overall carbohydrate intake. By being mindful of your choices and opting for lower-carb options, you can better manage your carbohydrate consumption and maintain a balanced diet.

5. **Legumes and beans**: When following a ketogenic diet, it is advisable to be cautious with legumes and beans such as lentils and chickpeas. These foods, while

nutritious, are relatively high in carbohydrates and may have an impact on the state of ketosis in the body. Therefore, it is recommended to limit or avoid their consumption to maintain the desired metabolic state.

6. **Unhealthy fats**: Unhealthy fats can harm our health. It is important to avoid trans fats, which are commonly found in processed snacks, fried foods, and margarine. Additionally, it is advisable to limit the intake of vegetable oils such as soybean, canola, and sunflower oil, as they have the potential to cause inflammation in the body. Being mindful of these fats can contribute to a healthier lifestyle.

7. **Sweetened condiments and sauces**: When following a Keto OMAD diet, be wary of sweetened condiments and sauces like ketchup, barbecue sauce, and salad dressings. These popular food items often contain added sugars and hidden carbs, which can quickly derail your weight loss goals. Instead, opt for homemade versions that are low in sugar and carbs, or search for keto-friendly alternatives available in stores. Stay vigilant and read labels carefully to maintain your ketogenic state.

8. **Alcohol**: It is important to limit or avoid alcoholic beverages as they are high in carbs which can hinder ketosis. It is best to opt for low-carb options like dry wines or spirits mixed with zero-calorie mixers.

However, it is crucial to note that alcohol consumption itself can temporarily stop the ketosis process, as the body prioritizes metabolizing alcohol over fats.

9. **Sugary and diet sodas**: It is essential to steer clear of sugary and diet sodas. These beverages can significantly impact blood sugar levels, leading to cravings and adversely affecting your dietary goals. Added sugar in regular sodas, and artificial sweeteners in diet sodas, can hinder your attempts to enter ketosis and promote fat-burning. With their negative impact on insulin sensitivity and glucose metabolism, it is prudent to avoid these drinks, instead opting for healthier alternatives such as water, herbal tea, or black coffee.

10. **Processed and packaged foods**: If you're following a Keto OMAD diet, avoid chips, crackers, and packaged snacks. These foods are loaded with hidden carbs, unhealthy fats, and additives that can derail your weight loss goals. Opt for fresh, whole foods instead to stay on track. Be vigilant and read food labels carefully to avoid sabotaging your progress. Remember, every food choice you make can make or break your success.

Remember, it's crucial to consult with a healthcare professional or registered dietitian before making any significant changes to your diet. They can provide personalized advice and guidance based on your specific health needs and goals.

Sample Recipes

Bacon-Wrapped Chicken Thighs

Ingredients:

- Chicken thighs
- Bacon
- Salt and pepper to taste

Instructions:

1. Preheat the oven to 375°F (190°C).

2. Wrap each chicken thigh with a slice of bacon.

3. Season the wrapped chicken thighs with salt and pepper.

4. Place the chicken thighs on a baking sheet and bake for 25-30 minutes or until the chicken is cooked through and the bacon is crispy.

Salmon with Asparagus

Ingredients:

- Salmon filets
- Asparagus
- Olive oil
- Salt and pepper to taste
- Lemon wedges for serving

Instructions:

1. Preheat the oven to 400°F (200°C).

2. Place the salmon filets and asparagus on a baking sheet.

3. Drizzle with olive oil and season with salt and pepper.

4. Bake for 12-15 minutes or until the salmon is cooked through and the asparagus is tender.

5. Serve with lemon wedges.

Cauliflower Fried Rice

Ingredients:

- 1 head of cauliflower, shredded or riced
- 2 tablespoons olive oil
- 1/2 onion, diced
- 1 cup frozen vegetables (peas, carrots, etc.)
- 2 cloves garlic, minced
- 2 eggs, beaten
- Salt and pepper to taste

Instructions:

1. Heat the olive oil in a skillet over medium-high heat.
2. Add the onion and sauté until softened, about 3 minutes.
3. Add the frozen vegetables and garlic and cook for 3 minutes, stirring occasionally.
4. Add the cauliflower rice and cook for 5 minutes, stirring occasionally.
5. Push the vegetables to one side of the skillet and add the beaten eggs.
6. Scramble the eggs until cooked through, stirring occasionally.

7. Stir together with the cooked vegetables and season with salt and pepper to taste.

8. Serve hot or cold.

Egg and Avocado Salad Lettuce Wraps

Ingredients:

- Romaine lettuce leaves
- Hard-boiled eggs
- Avocado
- Lemon juice
- Dijon mustard
- Salt and pepper to taste

Instructions:

1. Mash the hard-boiled eggs and avocado in a bow.

2. Add lemon juice, Dijon mustard, salt, and pepper. Mix well.

3. Spoon the egg & avocado salad onto individual romaine lettuce leaves.

4. Roll up the lettuce leaves and secure them with toothpicks if needed.

5. Serve as a refreshing and satisfying wrap.

Zucchini Noodles with Pesto and Grilled Chicken

Ingredients:

- Zucchini
- Grilled chicken breast
- Pesto sauce (homemade or store-bought)
- Cherry tomatoes (optional)
- Parmesan cheese (optional)

Instructions:

1. Using a spiralizer, create zucchini noodles from fresh zucchini.

2. Cook the zucchini noodles in a skillet over medium heat until tender, about 3-5 minutes.

3. Slice the grilled chicken breast into strips.

4. Toss the zucchini noodles with pesto sauce.

5. Top with grilled chicken and cherry tomatoes if desired.

6. Sprinkle grated Parmesan cheese for an extra flavor boost.

Steak with Creamy Garlic Mushrooms

Ingredients:

- Steak (such as ribeye or sirloin)
- Mushrooms
- Butter
- Garlic cloves
- Heavy cream
- Fresh parsley
- Salt and pepper to taste

Instructions:

1. Season the steak with salt and pepper.
2. Grill or pan-sear the steak to your desired doneness.
3. In a separate skillet, melt butter over medium heat.
4. Add minced garlic and sauté until fragrant.
5. Add sliced mushrooms and cook until they release their moisture and become golden brown.
6. Pour in heavy cream and simmer until the sauce thickens slightly.
7. Season with salt and pepper to taste.
8. Serve the steak topped with creamy garlic mushrooms and garnish with fresh parsley.

Taco Stuffed Bell Peppers

Ingredients:

- Bell peppers
- Ground beef or turkey
- Taco seasoning
- Shredded cheese
- Sour cream (optional)
- Salsa (optional)
- Guacamole (optional)

Instructions:

1. Preheat the oven to 350°F (180°C).

2. Cut the bell peppers in half and remove the seeds and membranes. Place them on a baking sheet lined with parchment paper.

3. Brown the ground beef or turkey in a skillet over medium heat, seasoning with taco seasoning as desired.

4. Divide the cooked meat among the bell pepper halves.

5. Top each bell pepper with shredded cheese.

6. Bake for 25 minutes or until the peppers are tender and the cheese is melted and bubbly.

7. Serve with sour cream, salsa, and guacamole if desired.

Creamy Spinach and Feta Stuffed Chicken

Ingredients:

- Chicken breasts
- Spinach
- Feta cheese
- Garlic powder
- Salt and pepper to taste

Instructions:

1. Preheat the oven to 350°F (180°C).

2. Cut a pocket in each chicken breast and stuff with the spinach and feta cheese.

3. Sprinkle it with garlic powder, salt, and pepper.

4. Place the stuffed chicken breasts on a baking sheet lined with parchment paper and bake for 25-30 minutes or until the chicken is cooked through.

5. Serve with a side salad, roasted vegetables, or mashed cauliflower for a delicious low-carb meal.

Cauliflower Crust Pizza

Ingredients:
- Cauliflower
- Mozzarella cheese
- Parmesan cheese
- Egg
- Pizza sauce
- Toppings of your choice (e.g., pepperoni, mushrooms, bell peppers)

Instructions:
1. Preheat the oven to 400°F (200°C).

2. Pulse cauliflower in a food processor until it has a rice-like consistency.

3. Microwave the cauliflower for 7 minutes or steam it until tender.

4. Transfer the cooked cauliflower to a large bowl and let it cool for 5 minutes.

5. Once cooled, add the mozzarella cheese, Parmesan cheese, and egg and mix until all ingredients are combined.

6. Press the cauliflower mixture into a greased pizza pan or baking sheet to create the crust.

7. Bake for 15 minutes or until the crust is golden brown and crisp around the edges.

8. Remove from the oven and spread with pizza sauce and desired toppings.

9. Return to the oven and bake for 15-20 minutes or until the cheese is melted and bubbly.

10. Slice into wedges and serve warm.

Shrimp Stir-Fry

Ingredients:

- Shrimp
- Low-sodium soy sauce or coconut aminos
- Sesame oil
- Garlic
- Ginger
- Broccoli florets
- Bell peppers
- Mushrooms
- Green onions

Instructions:

1. In a shallow bowl, mix the low-sodium soy sauce or coconut aminos and sesame oil.

2. Add the shrimp to the marinade and set aside for 15 minutes.

3. Heat a wok or large skillet over medium-high heat and add the garlic, ginger, broccoli florets, bell peppers, mushrooms, and green onions.

4. Stir-fry the vegetables for 4-5 minutes or until they are crisp and tender.

5. Add the marinated shrimp to the skillet and cook for another 5 minutes or until they are cooked through.

6. Serve over cauliflower rice or steamed quinoa for a complete meal.

Mediterranean Salad Paired with Charbroiled Chicken

Ingredients:

- Grilled chicken breast
- Romaine lettuce
- Cucumber
- Cherry tomatoes
- Red onion
- Kalamata olives
- Feta cheese
- Olive oil
- Lemon juice
- Dried oregano
- Salt and pepper to taste

Instructions:

1. Chop the grilled chicken breast into bite-sized pieces.

2. In a large bowl, combine chopped romaine lettuce, sliced cucumber, halved cherry tomatoes, thinly sliced red onion, and pitted kalamata olives.

3. Crumble feta cheese over the salad.

4. In a separate small bowl, whisk together olive oil, lemon juice, dried oregano, salt, and pepper to make the dressing.

5. Drizzle the dressing over the salad and toss to coat.

6. Top with grilled chicken before serving.

Zucchini and Bacon Egg Muffins

Ingredients:

- Zucchini
- Bacon
- Eggs
- Cheddar cheese
- Salt and pepper to taste

Instructions:

1. Preheat the oven to 375°F (190°C).
2. Grease a 12-cup muffin tin.
3. Chop the zucchini and bacon into small pieces.
4. Divide the zucchini and bacon evenly among the muffin cups.
5. Crack an egg into each cup and season with salt and pepper.
6. Sprinkle cheddar cheese over each muffin cup.
7. Bake for 15-20 minutes or until the eggs are cooked through and the cheese is melted and bubbly.
8. Serve warm with a side of sliced avocado and fresh fruit for a complete meal.

Lemon Garlic Shrimp Skewers

Ingredients:

- Shrimp
- Lemon
- Garlic cloves
- Olive oil
- Salt and pepper to taste

Instructions:

1. Preheat the grill to medium-high heat or preheat the broiler.

2. Soak wooden skewers in water for 10 minutes before grilling.

3. Thread shrimp onto the skewers and set aside.

4. In a bowl, combine lemon juice, minced garlic cloves, olive oil, salt, and pepper.

5. Drizzle the marinade over the shrimp skewers and let sit for 15 minutes.

6. Grill or broil the shrimp skewers for 5-7 minutes, flipping once, until they are cooked through and lightly charred.

7. Serve with a side salad or roasted vegetables for a delicious low-carb meal.

Caprese Stuffed Portobello Mushrooms

Ingredients:

- Portobello mushrooms
- Mozzarella cheese
- Tomato slices
- Fresh basil leaves
- Balsamic glaze
- Olive oil
- Salt and pepper to taste

Instructions:

1. Preheat the oven to 375°F (190°C).
2. Remove the stems from the portobello mushrooms and scoop out any gills.
3. Arrange the mushrooms on a baking sheet lined with parchment paper.
4. Top each mushroom cap with a slice of mozzarella cheese, followed by a tomato slice, and a few fresh basil leaves.
5. Drizzle with balsamic glaze and olive oil, and season with salt and pepper.

6. Bake for 15-20 minutes or until the cheese is melted and bubbly.

7. Serve with a side salad or roasted vegetables of your choice for a delicious low-carb meal.

Chocolate Avocado Mousse

Ingredients:

- Avocado
- Unsweetened cocoa powder
- Sugar-free sweetener (e.g., stevia, erythritol)
- Vanilla extract
- Almond milk or coconut milk

Instructions:

1. In a blender or food processor, combine ripe avocado flesh, unsweetened cocoa powder, sugar-free sweetener, vanilla extract, and a splash of almond milk or coconut milk.

2. Blend until smooth and creamy, adding more almond milk or coconut milk as needed for desired consistency.

3. Transfer the mousse to serving bowls or glasses.

4. Refrigerate for at least 30 minutes to allow it to set.

5. Serve chilled and enjoy!

7-Day Meal Plan

When following the Keto OMAD diet, it is important to make sure that your meals are balanced and contain all of the essential nutrients. Here is a sample 7-day meal plan to get you started:

Day 1

- Dinner: Bacon-Wrapped Chicken Thighs
- Side: Cauliflower Fried Rice

Day 2

- Dinner: Salmon with Asparagus
- Side: Egg & Avocado Salad Lettuce Wraps

Day 3

- Dinner: Zucchini Noodles with Pesto and Grilled Chicken

Day 4

- Dinner: Steak with Creamy Garlic Mushrooms
- Side: Creamy Spinach and Feta Stuffed Chicken

Day 5

- Dinner: Taco Stuffed Bell Peppers

Day 6

- Dinner: Shrimp Stir-Fry
- Side: Mediterranean Salad Paired with Charbroiled Chicken

Day 7

- Dinner: Cauliflower Crust Pizza
- Side: Zucchini and Bacon Egg Muffins

For dessert, you can enjoy Chocolate Avocado Mousse as a treat throughout the week.

Remember to adjust portion sizes and macronutrient ratios according to your specific needs and goals. Feel free to mix and match the meals based on your preferences. Enjoy your Keto OMAD meal plan!

Please note that this is just a sample meal plan based on the provided recipes, and you can adjust it to fit your personal preferences and nutritional needs. Make sure to consult with a healthcare professional or registered dietitian before starting any new diet or meal plan. Enjoy your Keto OMAD journey!

Conclusion

Congratulations! You've reached the end of our comprehensive guide to the Keto OMAD diet. By now, you should have a clear understanding of what this eating plan entails, how it can benefit your overall health, and some delicious recipe ideas to get you started. As you embark on this journey towards a healthier you, let's reflect on some key insights and encouragement to keep you motivated.

First and foremost, the Keto OMAD diet is not just a temporary fix or a quick weight loss solution; it's a lifestyle change. Adopting this way of eating requires dedication, discipline, and a long-term commitment to prioritizing your health.

Remember, Rome wasn't built in a day, and neither will your health transformation. Be patient with yourself, celebrate small victories along the way, and stay focused on your goals.

One of the most empowering aspects of the Keto OMAD diet is the control it gives you over your body and food choices. With one meal a day, you have the opportunity to plan and prepare nutrient-dense, satisfying meals that align with your dietary needs and preferences.

This level of control can help alleviate mindless eating habits, emotional eating, and unnecessary snacking. Embrace the freedom and empowerment that comes with making conscious, informed decisions about what you put into your body.

As you embark on your Keto OMAD journey, it's important to prioritize the quality of your food choices. Focus on consuming whole, unprocessed foods that are rich in healthy fats, moderate in protein, and low in carbohydrates.

Opt for organic produce, grass-fed meats, and wild-caught fish whenever possible. By nourishing your body with high-quality ingredients, you're providing it with the essential nutrients it needs to thrive.

It's also crucial to listen to your body's signals. Pay attention to hunger cues and satiety levels during your one meal a day. Remember, it's not about restricting yourself to the point of discomfort or deprivation; it's about finding a balance and nourishing your body adequately. If you find yourself feeling overly hungry or unsatisfied, consider adjusting your portion sizes or incorporating more filling foods into your meal.

Throughout your Keto OMAD journey, you may encounter challenges and setbacks. It's essential to approach these obstacles with a positive mindset and view them as learning opportunities rather than failures.

Stay curious, experiment with new recipes, and don't be afraid to seek support from online communities or friends who are also following this eating plan. Sharing experiences, insights, and successes can be incredibly motivating and enable you to stay on track.

As you progress on the Keto OMAD diet, remember that it's not just about weight loss. While shedding excess pounds may be a desired outcome for many, this way of eating offers numerous health benefits beyond the scale.

By reducing carb intake and increasing healthy fats, you can improve mental clarity, boost energy levels, control blood sugar, reduce inflammation, and enhance overall well-being. Celebrate non-scale victories and let them fuel your motivation on this path.

Self-care is crucial in any dietary journey. Prioritize sleep, manage stress, and incorporate physical activity into your routine. These lifestyle factors are key for optimal health and maximizing the positive effects of the Keto OMAD diet. Remember, you're nourishing your body, mind, and spirit.

In conclusion, the Keto OMAD diet offers a powerful tool for transforming your health and improving your quality of life. Embrace this lifestyle change with open arms, knowing that you have the power to take control of your nutrition and make choices that will positively impact your well-being. Stay motivated, seek support when needed, and celebrate every step forward on your journey to a healthier you. Remember, you've got this!

FAQs

What is the Keto OMAD diet?

The Keto OMAD diet combines the principles of the ketogenic diet with intermittent fasting. It involves consuming one meal a day within a specific time window while following a low-carbohydrate, high-fat eating plan.

What are the benefits of the Keto OMAD diet?

The Keto OMAD diet can promote weight loss, improve insulin sensitivity, increase energy levels, enhance mental clarity, and support overall metabolic health. It may also help regulate blood sugar levels and reduce inflammation.

Is the Keto OMAD diet suitable for everyone?

The Keto OMAD diet may not be suitable for everyone. Individuals with certain medical conditions, such as diabetes or eating disorders, should consult with a healthcare professional before starting this diet. Pregnant or breastfeeding women should also avoid it.

How do I start the Keto OMAD diet?

To start the Keto OMAD diet, educate yourself about the principles, macronutrient ratios, and recommended food choices. Gradually transition into intermittent fasting by extending your fasting hours each day until you reach your desired one-hour eating window.

What foods can I eat on the Keto OMAD diet?

The Keto OMAD diet focuses on high-quality fats, moderate protein, and low-carbohydrate foods. Examples include avocados, nuts, seeds, olive oil, fatty fish, poultry, eggs, non-starchy vegetables, and low-sugar fruits.

Can I snack during the fasting period on the Keto OMAD diet?

The Keto OMAD diet encourages only water, black coffee, or herbal tea during the fasting period. Snacking is generally discouraged outside the eating window to maintain the benefits of intermittent fasting and optimize fat burning.

How long should I follow the Keto OMAD diet?

The duration of following the Keto OMAD diet can vary based on individual needs and goals. Some people choose to adopt it as a long-term lifestyle, while others may follow it for a specific period to achieve their desired results. It's essential to listen to your body and adjust accordingly.

Resources and Helpful Links

Gough, S. M., Casella, A., Ortega, K. J., & Hackam, A. S. (2021). Neuroprotection by the ketogenic diet: Evidence and controversies. Frontiers in Nutrition, 8. https://doi.org/10.3389/fnut.2021.782657

Sharman, M. J., Kraemer, W. J., Love, D. M., Avery, N. G., Gómez, A. L., Scheett, T. P., & Volek, J. S. (2002). A ketogenic diet favorably affects serum biomarkers for cardiovascular disease in Normal-Weight men. Journal of Nutrition, 132(7), 1879–1885. https://doi.org/10.1093/jn/132.7.1879

Will One Meal A Day Slow My Metabolism| Dr. Berg. (n.d.). https://www.drberg.com/blog/will-one-meal-a-day-slow-my-metabolism#:~:text=How%20Effective%20Is%20OMAD%20with,burning%20and%20cellular%20repair%20processes.

Hamzic, H. (2021, December 13). OMAD and Keto: Benefits of combining the two - Hana Hamzic - medium. Medium. https://medium.com/@hanahamzic/omad-and-keto-benefits-of-combining-the-two-47d31c026cc4

Byakodi, R. (2021). OMAD Keto: Guide On Combining One Meal A Day With Keto. 21-Day Hero. https://21dayhero.com/omad-keto/

"Combining Keto With OMAD Diet Days And Occasional Extended Fasting Helped Me Lose 114 Pounds." (2020, July 9). Women's Health.

https://www.womenshealthmag.com/weight-loss/a33238453/keto-omad-diet-extended-fasting-weight-loss-success-story/

Robert. (2020). Keto OMAD – What is one meal a day? Addtoketo (UK). https://addtoketo.co.uk/keto-omad-what-is-one-meal-a-day/

www.ingramcontent.com/pod-product-compliance
Lightning Source LLC
LaVergne TN
LVHW021304080526
838199LV00090B/6005